ABC's of Nature's Best Herbal Recipes

Ombassa Sophera

ISBN-13: **978**-1497300842

ISBN-10: 1497300843

DEDICATION

This book is dedicated to my great-grandmother Mary Alvarez whose natural gifts of working alongside nature I am thankful to have inherited, to my Mom and Dad whose natural propensity for spiritual healing and emotional nurturing has gifted me with a legacy to love beyond all measure....I LOVE YOU ALL!

Disclaimer and Pledge

As a professional herbal practitioner of over 25 years, I have served my friends and family with natural remedies passed to me as a legacy by my ancestors and other teachers I've studied with along the way.

I now pass on to you, these age old recipes, for the sake of refreshing, balancing and energizing yourself for optimal wellbeing.

I make no claims about any medical condition regarding these herbal recipes, because indeed, be it a doctor, surgeon or herbal practitioner, the successful outcome of any of our treatments cannot with any certainty be predicted, let alone guaranteed. I encourage each one of you to begin to do your own research and study regarding all of the herbs and medicines you use.

Take full responsibility for your own health and well-being with this regard. I have included those herbal recipes that I am familiar with and have seen produce positive results.

Further, following USA law, the information in this material is attached to no medical claims.

I pledge that, I shall do all I can, using my knowledge of herbal medicines and natural treatments, to help you maintain your deserved state of well-being.

All the herbal tonics, poultices and baths are made with fresh herbs or dry herbs. Use organic, whole herbs when possible.

INTRODUCTION

Herbal Medicine provides each of us, a genuine anecdote to ingesting harsh drugs. Herbs gently nurture your body, while nourishing you back to a state of optimal health. Herbs have been used as food and medicine for thousands of years by every culture that has inhabited this planet. Our ancestors used herbs as a primary treatment for all health concerns, granting humankind with the ability to thrive and grow for many generations.

This book encompasses healing your whole body and inoculating your systems, guiding you towards ultimate health from the inside-out. The book provides a unique opportunity for you to create, a new and improved blueprint for living a wealth of health. This new blueprint is effectively achieved through mental and emotional exercises (intentional thoughts provided at the bottom of each recipe), the use of customized herbal blends and methods of energy balancing for the body, such as breathing and meditation exercises.

Too often, I see people tending to "own" their bodily imbalance-stating "my diabetes", "my high blood pressure", etc. It is for this specific reason that I have **deliberately** included **affirmative thoughts** with each recipe that uniquely speaks to each bodily imbalance. These affirmative thoughts reference what I know of the mindset or root cause of the illness or conditions experienced.
Great physicians, such as Imhotep and Hippocrates, who laid the foundation of medicine of today, also used this method of mind/body healing to complement the use of herbal medicine.

It is always important to do your own research of the herbs shared in these recipes before embarking on any new healing journey. Also, if you have placed yourself in a doctors' care, you should check with them as well, before using these recipes.

The recipes are not designed to in any fashion "fix" any condition you may be experiencing. What they will do, if put together properly, is assist you in your healing process, by refreshing and energizing your mind, body and spirit. I highly encourage you to utilize the poultices and baths along with tonics when balancing any issues with pain and circulation in particular, although the combination is exceptional with most all recipes.

Once you have made up your mind and set intention in your heart that your issue will be resolved, this is when the true healing begins.

Intuition is necessary when developing the proper measure for your tonic, as everyone's physiology differs.

Though we know that the perfect combination of herbs, foods and juices has a profound effect on the mental, emotional, and physical body, it has been scientifically proven that:

- Our bodies gathers and delivers the precise balance of neurochemicals that will reverse illness and cure disease. Your body thereby holds the innate capacity to heal itself.

- The substance of our thoughts and emotions directly and immediately impacts our biochemistry.

- We can consciously influence and direct the body's output through meditation and visualization techniques.

- Two people are not going to get the same results from the same remedy —customized herbal blends prepared especially for your energy can serve to bring positive results to any ailment or issue.

Finally, it is paramount to first examine your heart and mind about your health issue, before seeking to resolve it physically.

I trust you will find this book a wonderful resource for creating your new and improved blueprint for ultimate body systems.

Here's to your good health!

Ombassa Sophera

October 16, 2016

ACKNOWLEDGMENTS

Special thanks to all of my children, Devonna, Darin, Devin and Devita and their children: Nia, DJ, Nailah, Dalil and Dakari for your love and support as I completed the process of delivering this book, my gift to the world.

Thanks to my friends everywhere whose love I feel continually, for just being who you are in my life.

I LOVE YOU ALL !!!

DIRECTIONS FOR PREPARATIONS

HOLDING THE CORRECT INTENTION!

The recipe title and the intentional thoughts provided at the bottom of each recipe are designed to support you with your intention for a healthier body. As you prepare these formulas, it is very important to align your mind with the results you desire.

Holding the intentional thought in your mind is **most** important because every cell in the human body is connected to the mind. Every thought you think is received by each cell. Setting the correct intention while preparing the formula is akin to sending out an APB – All Points Bulletin to each cell. As you correct your thinking and align your mind with the Source of Perfect Health, your body, which is constantly rebuilding and repairing itself, will be energized with the power of your intention.

I am here to serve you further if you have questions or concerns: info@ombassa.com

DIRECTIONS FOR TONICS AND TEAS:

You will need:

Juicer

Lemon Juice Squeeze

A large pot

Glass gallon jugs

Extra-long spoon

3 gallons pure water (varies, discretion is recommended)

Unless otherwise specified in a tonic recipe, use **1 cup of each of leaf and flower herbs** and **½ cup of root, seed and bark herbs**. The roots, seeds and bark always go in the water first and should boil for at least 15-20 minutes over medium heat. Add the herbs and flowers and turn off the heat completely. Put the lid tightly on the pot and let steep for at least 1-6 hours before consuming. The longer it steeps the stronger the tonic will be.

When the recipe calls for lemons you will need to squeeze the juice of at least 12 lemons, more to your taste if you'd like. Where the recipe calls for any juice, always put in after the herbal mixture has completely cooled down.

The mixture should make at least three gallons which is the suggested dosage to begin your process with the tonics. Use your favorite healthy sweetener for your tonic if so desired (see list below).

Here are a few options:

- Agave
- Stevia
- Honey
- Pure Maple Syrup (B)

Always refrigerate after initial 24 hours of steeping. You may store it in refrigerator for up to two weeks. Your intuition/discretion is also necessary when deciding how long you continue to take herbal tonics for harmony and balance.

Of course, if you simply desire a refreshing drink to satisfy the moment you can use a tablespoon of leaf herb and a teaspoon of root and seed herbs.

DIRECTIONS FOR POULTICE:

What's in a Poultice?

Poultices are simply soaked herbs applied externally, typically to treat swelling, inflammation, congestion and pain. It is a really potent way to use herbs directly to a specific area-for a particular issue.

The constituents of the herbs are directly absorbed into our tissues through putting moistened herbs on the skin, with or without the use of a thin material, such as cheesecloth.

The poultice is high in concentration because of the ratio of herb to liquid-more herb than liquid.

Poultices are very useful for most anything that requires localized attention, getting faster results by being absorbed directly into the organ of the skin.

Basic Recipe Ingredients:

- Cheese Cloth or something similar

- Plastic Wrap
- Gauze or Bandages (in some cases)
- Herbal Blend
- Your preferred essential oils, if desired

According to your specific need, you may also add to recipe: slippery elm, bentonite, red clay, flax oil, castor oil, baking soda. Mix your ingredients together in a non-aluminum container (I use a wooden bowl and spoon), and use immediately.

METHODS OF APPLICATION:

The simple method of making poultice:

Pour hot water over chopped herbs in a reusable muslin bag. Apply just enough boiled water to moisten them so that they are not loose and runny.

Alternatively, the following steps are good for making a more intricate poultice to apply to issues such as chest congestion and coughing.

- Chop herbs then moistened with either oils (castor or linseed), apple-cider vinegar or hot water.
- Mix the herbs (and essential oils if desired) with clay, whole wheat flour or cornmeal, to hold it together. The proportion should be 1 part herb to 3 parts vehicle.
- Spread the mixture on a warm, moist cloth or gauze and fold the ends and sides over.

When applying with moist cloth or gauze it serves two purposes: first, it ensures that small particles of herbs can't get into an open wound; secondly, it allows the poultice to be easily lifted off when finished without having to wipe bits of herb off the skin. This is important because when you remove the poultice you want any remaining herb infused liquid to dry on the skin. Use the minimum amount of layers of gauze to both prevent bits of herb from getting through, yet receive the properties of the herbal blend well. The number of layers will depend on the thickness of the gauze.

When applying the poultice, completely cover an area a bit larger than the area with moistened herbs using a spoon, press down on them so that there is adequate contact with the skin.

Because the skin is normally water-proof, to get the components of the herbs in the poultice to penetrate the skin, it must be hydrated to eliminate its water-proof characteristics. To accomplish this, it's necessary for the entire area designated for the poultice to remain moist. The object is to not allow the skin to breathe, only accept the components of your blend.

To accelerate this process, it is necessary that the poultice be applied as hot as can be tolerated and remain warm for the duration of the application. The longer the poultice is in contact with the skin, the more hydrated our skin becomes and the better the penetration. Usually a minimum of 30 minutes, but 1-4 or more hours may sometime be necessary, depending on the severity of the condition being treated.

To facilitate the hydration of the skin it is sometimes best to wrap the poultice in plastic so that the skin remains in complete contact with herb infused liquid from the poultice. Most types of plastic wrap are made of polyethylene which isn't known to leach any toxic chemicals will work for this. After wrapping the poultice I recommend pushing down on it once more to make sure there is good contact with the skin and no air spaces between the plastic and the herbs.

This whole process must be done as quickly as possible so that the herbs are still hot. Once the poultice has been wrapped in plastic it is necessary to cover it with a towel or something similar to help insulate it to keep it warm. If is going to be applied for a long period of time it may be necessary to apply a hot compress over the plastic. A cloth soaked in hot water that has been wrung out so that it isn't dripping will do. The cloth can be reheated periodically when it cools down. If the area where we need to apply the poultice isn't too large, a hot water bottle will also work and is more convenient than using a compress.

You may choose to apply a poultice for 45-60 minutes twice per day, or decide to leave on 4-6 at a time, intuition/discretion is yours to use here. When using gauze, the whole thing will lift off very easily. After removing the poultice, the skin will be moist, don't wipe this off. Let it dry completely before covering the area with anything.

Once dry, the process is complete. You may bandage the area, if necessary, or cover it in some other way. You may also apply an ointment or liniment to the area, if appropriate, to further assist the healing process.

Which herbs used, how often and how long to apply a poultice will depend on the situation, but the basic elements of applying a poultice will always be the same.

POULTICES SPECIFIC TO INJURIES:

Place fresh herbs in either food processor or blender, along with 1/2 cup of water and purée on High level until it becomes liquid.

Pour into bowl and add a handful of flour (or any binding agent, I like clay) and stir it until mixture binds slightly as a paste. (add more binding agent as needed)

Use a rubber spatula to scrape paste onto clean cloth folded in half lengthwise.

Fold edges over to slightly contain mixture, but leave enough exposed to come in direct contact with affected injured area.

Leave poultice on at least an hour up until 4 hours or as needed. Discretion is also necessary here.

ABC's of Nature's Best Herbal Recipes

DIRECTIONS FOR BATHS:

What's in Herbal Baths and Foot Soaks

An aromatic bath or foot soak is one of the simplest and most delightful forms of herbal therapy. Just the thought of soaking in hot water is relaxing, and then when you add herbs or essential oils to this experience it becomes a sensual treat that is sure to soothe, rejuvenate and stimulate the mind, body and spirit.

These herbal blends are easy to use dried herbs and flowers, sometimes in combination with essential oils, salts and other oils for bath and foot soaks. These aromatic preparations are packaged and can be combined with other spa items such as a nail brush, luffa, cotton washcloth or towel, or whatever you dream up for your relaxing and invigorating experience (candles are a nice added effect).

Each individual may react differently, so be sure to do a patch test on the skin before using the soaks, especially if you have not used this particular blend before. Apply a small amount of the blend, dissolved in a little water if needed, to the inner part of the elbow and wait a few hours to see if any redness or itching develops.

Note: Essential oils are concentrated and very strong, they should be added to carrier oils before adding them to the tub or applying on the skin. Most essential oils should not be applied directly to the skin. Many essential oils are not safe for use by pregnant or nursing women. Do your research carefully if you or anyone using the products (expectant mother or others) could be at risk of an adverse reaction.

You will need:

1 part Epsom salt

1 part Baking soda

1 part Himalayan salt

4 parts preferred herbal blend

Mix together all ingredients thoroughly then store in an airtight container. Use 3 to 6 tablespoons of blend per gallon of water used. Water temperature should be as warm as your body tolerates for optimal relief. Steep your herbs in 1 gallon of hot water for at least 30 minutes before using.

If you have essential oils that are already working for you, you may add this to your bath also. Marbles or smooth river rocks can be added to the bottom of the foot basin to rub feet over while they're soaking, it is quite soothing!

Additional note...
Always use the discernment from yourself and your physician in whether to use a particular blend and do your own research if there is any doubt. These blends are simply here to assist you on your wellbeing journey. Enjoy!

TABLE OF CONTENTS

DISCLAIMER AND PLEDGE   IV

INTRODUCTION   V

DIRECTIONS FOR PREPARATIONS   VIII

DIRECTIONS FOR TONICS AND TEAS: ix

DIRECTIONS FOR POULTICE: x

DIRECTIONS FOR BATHS: xiv

ACKNOWLEDGMENTS   VII

███████   7

ACIDITY   8

ACNE   9

ADDICTIONS   10

ADRENALS   11

ALLERGIES   12

APPETITE   13

ANOREXIA   14

ANTI-BACTERIAL   15

ANTIBIOTIC   16

ANTI-COAGULANT 17

ANTI-DEPRESSANT 18

ANTI-INFLAMMATORY 19

ANTIOXIDANT 20

ANTI-SPASMODIC 21

ANTI-VIRAL 22

ANTISEPTIC 23

ANXIETY 24

ARTHRITIS 25

ATHLETE'S FOOT 26

BAD BREATH 27

BEDWETTING 28

BLADDER 29

BLOOD PURIFIER 30

BLOOD PRESSURE – HIGH 31

BLOOD PRESSURE – LOW 32

BOILS 33

BONE HEALTH 34

BRAIN 35

BREAST MILK – DECREASE 36

BREAST MILK – INCREASE 37

BRONCHITIS 38

BRUISES 39

CHILLS 40

CIRCULATION 41

COLIC 42

COLON CLEANSE 43

CONGESTION 44

COUGHS 45

CRAMPS 46

DIARRHEA 47

DIGESTIVE TRACT 48

DIURETIC 49

DRY SKIN	**50**
EAR INFECTION	**51**
EDEMA	**52**
ENERGY	**53**
EXHAUSTION	**54**
EYES	**55**
FEMALE WELL-BEING	**56**
FERTILITY	**57**
FLU	**58**
FUNGAL INFECTIONS	**59**
GOUT	**60**
HAY FEVER	**61**
HEADACHES	**62**
HEARTBURN	**63**
HEMORRHOIDS	**64**
HIGH CHOLESTEROL	**65**
HORMONAL BALANCE	**66**
IMMUNE SYSTEM	**67**

IMPOTENCE 68

INCONTINENCE 69

IBS(Irritable Bowel Syndrome) 70

JAUNDICE 71

JOINTS 72

KIDNEYS 73

LIVER 74

MALE WELL-BEING 75

MOTION SICKNESS 76

MOUTH/GUMS 77

NAUSEA 78

NERVES 79

NIGHT SWEATS 80

NOSEBLEEDS 81

PMS 82

PAIN	83
PARASITES	84
PREGNANCY TEA	85
PROSTATE	86
RASHES	87
SCALP ISSUES	88
SCARS	89
SEXUAL ORGANS	90
SINUS	91
STOMACH	92
THROAT	93
THYROID	94
TONSILLITIS	95
TORN LIGAMENTS	96
URINARY INFECTION	97
VARICOSE VEINS	98
WEIGHT LOSS	99
ABOUT THE AUTHOR	100

RECIPES

ACIDITY

1 cup Chamomile Flowers
1 cup Fennel Seed
½ cup Slippery Elm Bark
½ cup Parsley Leaf
1 cup Marshmallow Root
1 cup Spearmint Leaf
2 cups Peppermint Leaf
½ cup Anise Seed
¼ cup Bay Leaves

"I am balanced with life."

ACNE

1 pint Aloe Juice (non-acidic)
1 cup Calendula Flowers
¼ Lavender Flowers
1 cup Walnut Leaf
1 cup Witch Hazel Leaf
½ cup Burdock Root
1 cup Milk Thistle Leaf
1 cup Buchu Leaf
¼ cup Chamomile Flowers
¼ cup Whole Cloves
¼ cup Comfrey Root
½ cup Parsley Root

"I accept who I am in every way."

ADDICTIONS

1 cup Lemon Balm
2 cups Milk Thistle Seed
1 cup Agrimony
½ cup Licorice Root
½ cup Red Clover Leaf
½ cup Burdock Root
1 cup Dandelion Leaf
½ cup Yellow Dock Root
1 cup Peppermint Leaf
½ cup Kudzu Root
¼ cup Wormwood Leaf
½ cup Kava Kava Root
½ cup St John's Wort Leaf

"I am free, nothing has a hold over me."

ADRENALS

½ Licorice Root
1 cup Sarsaparilla Root
1 cup Bladderwrack Leaf
½ cup Irish Moss
½ cup Ginger Root
1 cup Astragalus Leaf
2 tbl Cayenne Pepper
1 cup Rose Hips Extract

"I take very special care of me."

ALLERGIES

1 cup Chamomile Flowers
1 cup Echinacea Leaf
1 cup Stinging Nettles Leaf
1 cup Plantain Leaf
¼ cup Butterbur Leaf
½ cup Astralagus Leaf
¼ cup Ephedra Leaf
½ cup Thyme Leaf

"I claim my Divine power within."

APPETITE

1 cup Ginger Root
2 cup Blessed Thistle Leaf
2 cups Peppermint Leaf
1 tbl Nutmeg
1 tsp Cinnamon
1 Quart Fresh Pressed Apple Juice
12 Lemons

"I bless the healing power of food."

ANOREXIA

¼ cup Cardamom Seed Juice
1 bulb Garlic
½ cup Ginger Root
½ cup Thyme Leaf
2 cups Alfalfa Leaf
1 cup Yarrow Leaf
1 cup Peppermint Leaf
½ cup Fennel Seed
½ cup Hyssop Leaf
½ cup Dandelion Leaf
½ cup Wormwood Leaf
½ cup Fenugreek Seed
½ cup Lemon Balm Leaf
½ cup Chamomile Flowers

"I allow myself to enjoy all of life's delights today!"

ANTI-BACTERIAL

½ cup Oregon Grape Root
½ cup Turmeric Root
1 cup Calendula Flowers
¼ cup Cinnamon Bark
½ cup Lavender Flowers
¼ cup Marjoram Leaf
1 cup Witch Hazel Leaf
1 cup White Oak Bark
½ cup Clove Bud

"Only purity lives within me."

ANTIBIOTIC

1 cup Goldenseal Leaf
½ cup Bladderwrack Leaf
1 cup Buchu Leaf
1 cup Echinacea Leaf
½ cup Echinacea Root
1 cup Alfalfa Leaf
¼ cup Rosemary Leaf
¼ cup Sage
Juice bulb of Garlic
Juice 12 Lemons

"I purify my mind and my heart with love."

ANTI-COAGULANT

¼ cup Cayenne Pepper
1 cup Pennywort Leaf
½ cup Turmeric Root
1 cup Alfalfa Leaf
½ cup Angelica Leaf
¼ cup Anise Seed
¼ cup Arnica Leaf
½ cup Celery Seed
Juice bulb of Garlic

"My life force flows freely."

ANTI-DEPRESSANT

¼ cup Damiana Leaf
½ cup Ginseng Leaf
½ cup Lady's Slipper Leaf
½ cup Saffron Leaf
½ cup Ginkgo Leaf
¼ cup Jasmine Flowers
¼ cup Lavender Flowers
¼ cup Lemon Verbena leaf
1 cup Oat Straw Leaf
½ cup Rosemary Leaf
¼ cup St John's Wort Leaf

"I am worthy of a beautiful life, I accept it now."

ANTI-INFLAMMATORY

1 cup Basil Leaf

1 cup Bergamot Leaf

½ cup Chamomile Flowers

½ cup Turmeric Powder

1 cup Red Clover Leaf

1 cup Echinacea Leaf

½ cup Ginger Root

½ cup Rosemary Leaf

1 cup Yarrow Leaf

1 cup Sorrel Blossoms

½ cup Sheep Sorrel Leaf

"I release the hurt, anger and transmute it into love."

ANTIOXIDANT

20 Lemons
½ cup Turmeric Root
Pinch of Cayenne Pepper
1 cup Echinacea Root
1 cup Echinacea Leaf
½ cup Goldenseal Root
1 cup Goldenseal Leaf 1
cup Elder Berries
1 cup Sorrel Blossoms

"My love is a POWERFUL defense for anything I may encounter in life."

ANTI-SPASMODIC

¼ cup Anise Seed
½ cup Basil Leaf
¼ cup Cardamom Seed
1 cup Chamomile Flowers
¼ Cinnamon Bark
¼ cup Cloves Bud
½ cup Lemon Thyme Leaf
½ cup Lemon Verbena Leaf
½ cup Marjoram Leaf
½ Lemon Balm Leaf
¼ cup Rosemary Leaf
½ cup St John's Wort Leaf
1 cup Yarrow Leaf

"I relax and let flow happen."

ANTI-VIRAL

Juice 2 bulbs Garlic
1 cup Oregano Leaf
1 cup Astralagus Leaf
1 cup Echinacea Root
1 cup Schizandra Berries
1 cup Elderberry
½ cup Echinacea Leaf
½ cup Licorice Root
½ cup Buchu Leaf
½ cup Goldenrod Leaf
½ cup Olive Leaf
¼ cup Juniper Berries
¼ cup Lemon Balm Leaf
¼ cup Shitake Mushroom
¼ cup Ginger Root
¼ cup Goldenseal Leaf
¼ cup St John's Wort
½ cup Rose Hips Fruit

"I trust the Universal supply."

ANTISEPTIC

1 cup Bergamot Leaf
1 cup Calendula Flowers
1 cup Witch Hazel Leaf
½ cup White Oak Bark
½ cup Cloves Bud
½ cup Ginger Root
¼ Lavender Flowers
1 cup Rose Hips Fruit
1 cup Yarrow Leaf

"I am at peace with love for who I am."

ANXIETY

1 cup Kava Kava Root
½ cup Ginseng Leaf
½ cup Valerian Root
½ cup Lemon Balm Leaf
1 cup Catnip Leaf
¼ cup St John's Wort Leaf
1 cup Chamomile Flowers
¼ cup Lavender Flowers
½ cup Alfalfa Leaf
1 cup Peppermint Leaf
1 cup Oat Straw

"I no longer give my peace away to_____.(fill in your issue)"

ARTHRITIS

1 cup Alfalfa Leaf
1 cup Black Cohosh Leaf
1 cup Bladderwrack Leaf
¼ cup Oregano Leaf
3 tbls Cayenne Pepper
1 cup Celery Leaf
1 cup Red Clover Leaf
½ cup Comfrey Root
½ cup Devils Claw Leaf
¼ cup Ginger Root
½ cup Parsley Leaf
¼ cup Nettles Leaf
¼ cup Turmeric Root
¼ cup Burdock Root
¼ cup Wild Yam Root
½ cup White Willow Bark

"My joy has moved my heart to sing."

ATHLETE'S FOOT

1 cup Buchu Leaf
1 cup Calendula Flowers
½ cup Olive Leaf
1 cup Pau D Arco Leaf
½ cup Goldenseal Root
1 cup Witch Hazel Leaf
1 cup White Oak Bark
¼ cup Thyme Leaf
1 cup Goldenseal Leaf
1 cup Echinacea Root
1 cup Echinacea Leaf

"The path is clear for my new walk."

BAD BREATH

½ cup Clove Bud
½ cup Anise Seed
½ cup Caraway Seed
½ cup Fennel Seed
½ cup Coriander Seed
½ cup Cardamom Seed
1 cup Parsley Leaf
1 cup Peppermint Leaf
½ cup Spearmint Leaf
¼ cup Wintergreen Leaf

"I allow a new attitude of sweetness"

BEDWETTING

½ cup Oak Bark
1 cup Catmint Leaf
½ cup Uva Ursi Leaf
½ cup Horsetail Leaf
1 cup Mullein Flowers
½ cup Plantain Leaf
1 quart 100% Cranberry Juice
1 cup Corn Silk
Honey to taste

"I am supported and secure in love."

BLADDER

1 cup Juniper Berries
1 cup Buchu Leaf
1 cup Celery Seeds
½ cup Fennel Seeds
1 cup Parsley Leaf
¼ cup Borage Leaf
1 cup Corn Silk
1 cup Uva Ursi Leaf
1 Quart Cranberry Juice
½ cup Dandelion Leaf
1 cup Goldenrod Leaf
½ cup Echinacea Leaf
½ cup Horsetail Leaf
¼ cup Lemon Balm Leaf

"Releasing toxic emotions is easy for me now."

BLOOD PURIFIER

1 cup Burdock Root
1 cup Basil Leaf
1 cup Echinacea Root
1 cup Echinacea Leaf
1 cup Red Clover Leaf
1 cup Alfalfa Leaf
½ cup Dandelion Root
½ cup Yellowdock Leaf

"My flow of life is pure."

BLOOD PRESSURE – HIGH

1 cup Gingko Leaf

1 cup Hawthorn Berries

¼ cup Siberian Ginseng Root

Juice Garlic (bulb)

1 cup Maitake Mushroom

1 cup Olive Leaf

½ cup Basil Leaf

½ cup Celery Seeds

1 cup Yarrow Leaf

"I now choose to resolve deep-seated emotional issues."

BLOOD PRESSURE – LOW

1 cup Rosemary Leaf
1 cup Motherwort Leaf
1 cup Hawthorn Berries
½ cup Ginger Root
1 cup Ginseng Root
1 cup Siberian Ginseng Root
½ cup Scotch Broom Leaf or Flower
½ cup Indian Spikeard Leaf
1 cup Nettle Leaf

"Nothing's gonna get me down."

BOILS

Juice bulb of Garlic
Juice 12 Lemons
1 cup Goldenseal Leaf
½ cup Bladderwrack Leaf
1 cup Buchu Leaf
1 cup Echinacea Leaf
½ cup Echinacea Root
1 cup Alfalfa Leaf
¼ cup Rosemary Leaf
¼ cup Sage Leaf

"I am love, joy and peace."

BONE HEALTH

1 cup Comfrey Root
1 Quart Aloe Juice
1 cup Peppermint Leaf
1 cup Horsetail Leaf
¼ cup Turmeric Root
½ cup Cactus Leaf
½ cup Marshmallow Leaf

"I allow wholeness."

BRAIN

1 cup Gotu Kola Leaf

1 cup Asian Ginseng Root

1 cup Siberian Ginseng Root

1 cup Guarana Berry

1 cup Gingko Leaf

½ cup Rosemary Leaf

1 cup Raspberry Leaf

1 cup Peppermint Leaf

½ cup Pennywort Leaf

"I enhance my cells and use every part of my brain."

BREAST MILK – DECREASE

1 cup Peppermint Leaf
1 cup Spearmint Leaf
1 cup Parsley Leaf
½ cup Red Raspberry Leaf
1 cup Chickweed Leaf
½ cup Black Walnut Leaf
1 cup Yarrow Leaf
¼ cup Lemon Balm Leaf

"I flow my love to other areas of my child's life."

BREAST MILK – INCREASE

1 cup Blessed Thistle Leaf

1 cup Fenugreek Seed

1 cup Fennel Seed

½ cup Anise Seed

¼ cup Coriander Seed

¼ cup Spearmint Leaf

¼ cup Lemongrass Leaf

¼ cup Lemon Verbena Leaf

½ cup Marshmallow Leaf

1 cup Nettles Leaf

½ cup Alfalfa Leaf

½ cup Hops Flowers

¼ cup Caraway Seeds

"I increase my flow of love to my newborn."

BRONCHITIS

½ cup Anise Seed

½ cup Cardamom Seed

1 cup Red Clover Leaf

1 cup Comfrey Leaf

1 cup Echinacea Leaf

1 cup Elderflower Leaf

½ cup Thyme Leaf

½ cup Mullein Leaf

¼ cup Anise Seed

½ cup Licorice Root

½ cup Nettle Leaf

¼ cup Caraway Seed

½ cup Coltsfoot Leaf

¼ cup Elecampane Leaf

½ cup Eucalyptus Leaf

½ cup Fennel Seed

½ cup Gingko Leaf

½ cup Honeysuckle Leaf

"My family environment is healing peacefully through me."

BRUISES

1 cup Bilberry Leaf

1 cup Stinging Nettle Leaf

1 cup Oat Straw

½ cup Ginger Root

1 cup Comfrey Root

½ cup Comfrey Leaf

¼ cup Lavender Flowers

½ cup Marjoram Leaf

1 cup Calendula Flowers

"Love is all I want, need and have. I'm now free to cherish me."

CHILLS

1 cup Echinacea Leaf
½ cup Echinacea Root
1 cup Ginger Root
¼ cup Turmeric Root
3 tbl Cayenne Pepper
½ cup Licorice Root
½ cup Burdock Root
½ cup Chamomile Flowers
½ cup Cleavers Leaf/Stems
1 cup Alfalfa Leaf
12 Squeezed Lemons

"I desire to stay in the present moment."

CIRCULATION

1 cup Ginger Root
1 cup Ginkgo Leaf
¼ cup Cayenne Pepper
1 cup Rosemary Leaf
½ cup Gotu Kola Leaf
½ cup Rosemary Leaf
1 cup Yarrow Leaf
1 cup Hawthorn Berries
1 Whole Bulb Garlic
¼ cup Horse Chestnut Leaf

"I live my truth and circulate my joy freely."

COLIC

1 cup Bay Leaves
½ cup Anise Seed
½ cup Caraway Seed
½ cup Cardamom Seed
1 cup Catmint Leaf
1 cup Chamomile Flowers
½ cup Fennel Seed
½ cup Lemon Grass Leaf
½ cup Lemon Verbena Leaf
1 cup Lemon Balm Leaf
1 cup Peppermint Leaf
1 cup Rose Hips Fruit
1 cup Strawberry Leaf

"I am completely safe. I love being here."

*This mixture needs to be diluted ten parts or more of pure water to one part herbal mixture for babies. Discretion is always necessary here, mothers need always taste the mixture first, to see if they are satisfied with the strength.
Nursing mothers can feed this formula through their milk.

COLON CLEANSE

1 cup Blessed Thistle Leaf
1 cup Fenugreek Seed
1 cup Fennel Seed
½ cup Cape Aloe Powder
1 cup Cascara Sagrada Leaf
½ cup Senna Leaf
½ cup Anise Seed
¼ cup Coriander Seed
1 cup Peppermint Leaf
¼ cup Spearmint Leaf
¼ cup Lemongrass Leaf
¼ cup Lemon Verbena Leaf
½ cup Marshmallow Leaf
1 cup Nettles Leaf
½ cup Alfalfa Leaf
¼ cup Caraway Seed

"I willingly release all stuck patterns."

CONGESTION

½ cup Horseradish Root
½ cup Ginger Root
20 Squeezed Lemons
1 cup Comfrey Root
1 cup Elecampane Root
1 cup Slippery Elm Bark
½ cup Eucalyptus Leaf
1 cup Horehound Leaf
1 cup Hyssop Leaf
½ cup Pleurisy Root
1 cup Mullein Flowers
1 cup Coltsfoot Leaf
¼ cup Cayenne Pepper
1 cup Peppermint Leaf
¼ cup Spearmint Leaf

"I allow my emotions to flow free into complete release."

COUGHS

1 cup Wild Cherry Bark

1 Pint Raw Honey

20 Squeezed Lemons

1 cup Slippery Elm Bark

1 cup Peppermint Leaf

1 cup Elderflower Leaf

½ cup Ginger Root

½ cup Elecampane Root

½ cup Slippery Elm Bark

½ cup Eucalyptus Leaf

1 cup Horehound Leaf

¼ cup Hyssop Leaf

¼ cup Pleurisy Root

1 cup Lemon Thyme Leaf

1 cup Mullein Flowers

"I speak distinctly, my wishes and I am clearly heard."

CRAMPS

1 cup Cramp Bark
1 cup Peppermint Leaf
1 cup Alfalfa Leaf
½ cup Valerian Root
1 cup Skullcap Leaf
½ cup Yarrow Leaf
1 cup Chamomile Flowers
½ cup Calamus Leaf
½ cup Lavender Flowers
¼ cup Cinnamon Bark
¼ cup Red Peony Root
½ cup Chinese Motherwort Leaf
½ cup Chinese Angelica Leaf

"I release into the process of life. Life happens well for me."

DIARRHEA

1 cup Agrimony Leaf
1 cup Bilberry Leaf
2 tbl Cayenne Pepper
¼ cup Fenugreek Seed
1 cup Peppermint Leaf
1 cup Marshmallow Leaf
½ cup Pau D Arco Leaf
1 cup Raspberry Leaf
½ cup Strawberry Leaf
2 tbl Nutmeg

"I accept my life as it is right now"

DIGESTIVE TRACT

½ cup Anise Seed
1 cup Parsley Leaf
1 cup Peppermint Leaf
½ cup Caraway Seed
½ cup Cardamom Seed
½ cup Fennel Seed
1 cup Marshmallow Leaf
1 cup Slippery Elm Bark
1 cup Chamomile Flowers
1 cup Lemon Balm Leaf
½ cup Gentian Root
½ cup Oregon Grape Root
½ cup Skullcap Leaf
½ cup Goldenseal Root
1 cup Wormwood Leaf

"With ease I assimilate what life has for me."

DIURETIC

1 cup Celery Seed
1 cup Corn Silk
1 cup Parsley Leaf
1 cup Stinging Nettle Leaf
¼ cup Hops Flower
¼ cup Fennel Seed
¼ cup Chicory Mint Leaf
½ cup Yarrow Leaf
¼ cup Goldenseal Root
½ cup Dandelion Leaf
1 cup Nettle Leaf
½ cup Marshmallow Leaf
1 cup Spearmint Leaf
1 cup Artichoke Leaf
¼ cup Chamomile Flowers

"I feel lifted, light and balanced."

DRY SKIN

1 cup Borage Leaf
1 cup Dandelion Leaf
1 cup Milk Thistle Seed
1 cup Calendula Flowers
½ cup Lady's Mantle Flowers
1 cup Marshmallow Leaf
1 cup Lemon Balm Leaf
½ cup Clary Sage Leaf

"I feel comfortable in my skin."

EAR INFECTION

1 cup Echinacea Leaf

1 cup Elder Flowers

1 Whole Bulb Garlic

1 cup Alfalfa Leaf

1 cup Mullein Flowers

1 cup Goldenseal Leaf

½ cup Goldenseal Root

1 cup Olive Leaf

"I clear my ear to hear with love"

EDEMA

1 cup Celery Seed
1 cup Raspberry Leaf
2 cups Corn Silk
1 cup Cleavers
1 cup Parsley Leaf
½ cup Fennel Seed
1 cup Alfalfa Leaf
1 cup Juniper Berries
½ cup Uva Ursi Leaf
1 cup Dandelion Leaf

"For my highest healing, I let of_____."(Fill in the blank)

ENERGY

½ cup Ashwagandha

1 cup Yerba Mate Leaf

¼ cup Korean Ginseng Root

½ Siberian Ginseng

¼ cup Ginger Root

½ cup Green Tea

½ cup Ginkgo Root

1 cup Alfalfa Leaf

"I claim my massive measure of God-given energy."

EXHAUSTION

2 cups Alfalfa Leaf
1 cup Oat Straw
½ cup Peppermint Leaf
½ cup Rosemary Leaf
1 cup Gotu Kola Leaf
1 cup Guarana Leaf
2 tbls Cayenne Pepper
1 cup Ginkgo Leaf
1 cup Siberian Ginseng Leaf
½ cup Ashwaganda Leaf
½ cup Astragalus Leaf
½ cup Stinging Nettle Leaf
¼ cup Reishi Mushroom

"I am rejuvenating now."

EYES

½ cup Fennel Seeds
1 cup Eyebright Leaf
½ cup Ginkgo Root
¼ cup Milk Thistle Seeds
¼ cup Saffron Powder
1 cup Bilberry Leaf
½ cup Anise Seed
1 cup Passionflower

"I can see clearly now."

*Additional info for eyes: Bentonite Clay, Chickweed and Fennel poultice will work wonders in both removing toxins and soothing the eyes. Eyebright still works wonders as an eyewash.

FEMALE WELL-BEING

1 cup False Unicorn Root
1 cup Damiana Leaf
2 cups Red Raspberry Leaf
½ cup Fo-Ti Root
½ cup Wild Yam Root
1 cup Catnip Leaf
1 cup Echinacea Leaf
½ cup Hyssop Leaf
¼ cup Licorice Root
½ cup Elder Flower
¼ cup Ginger Root
¼ cup Lemon Grass
½ cup Yarrow Leaf
¼ cup Cinnamon Bark
3 tbl Clove Bud

"I choose love, abundance, peace, clarity and wealth of health."

FERTILITY

1 cup Red Raspberry Leaf

1 cup Dong Quai Root

½ cup False Unicorn Leaf

½ cup Damiana Leaf

¼ cup Oat Straw

1 cup Nettle Leaf

¼ cup Dandelion Leaf

¼ cup Alfalfa Leaf

¼ cup Red Clover Leaf

¼ cup Maca Root

¼ cup Vitex/Chaste Tree Berries

"I now lay fertile ground for new life."

FLU

1 cup Mullein Leaf
1 cup Sage Leaf
1 cup Elder Berry
1 cup Slippery Elm Bark
1 Whole Bulb Garlic
1 ½ Echinacea Leaf
1 cup Yarrow Leaf
½ cup Ginger Root
1 cup Buchu Leaf
½ cup Goldenseal Root
½ cup Licorice Root
½ cup Lemon Balm Leaf
½ cup Oregano Leaf
½ cup Thyme Leaf

"I claim my individual right to remain positive."

FUNGAL INFECTIONS

½ cup Myrrh Gum
½ cup Black Walnut Bark
¼ cup Clove Bud
¼ cup Cinnamon
1 Quart Aloe Juice
1 cup Turmeric Root
1 cup Echinacea Leaf
½ cup Marigold Flowers
1 Whole Bulb Garlic
¼ cup Cayenne Pepper

"I release the past, it has no power over me now.
"I release and let the present moment rule."

GOUT

2 quarts Cherry Juice
2 cups Parsley Leaf
1 cup Stinging Nettle Leaf
½ cup Cleavers Leaf/Stems
¼ cup Coriander Seeds
1 cup Red Clover Leaf
½ cup Fennel Seed
½ cup Devils Claw Root
1 cup Celery Seed
1 cup Artichoke Leaf
½ cup Gravel Root (Kidneywort)
½ cup Turmeric Root
1 cup Alfalfa Leaf

"I submit to patience and joy."

HAY FEVER

1 cup Butterbur Leaf
1 cup Stinging Nettles Leaf
½ cup Ginkgo Leaf
¼ cup Cinnamon Bark
1 cup Elderflowers
¼ cup Ephedra Powder
½ cup Eyebright Leaf
½ cup Ginkgo Leaf
1 cup Peppermint Leaf
½ cup Reishi Mushrooms
¼ cup Rosemary Leaf
1 cup Violet Leaf

"I am safe within the flow of my life."

HEADACHES

1 cup Chamomile Flowers
½ Goldenseal Leaf
1 cup Licorice Root
1 cup Marshmallow Leaf
1 cup Slippery Elm Bark
½ cup Kava Kava Root
½ cup White Willow Bark
½ cup Turmeric Root
1 cup Peppermint Leaf

"I ease my body into peace and calm."

HEARTBURN

½ cup Slippery Elm Bark
1 cup Fennel Seed
½ cup Anise Seed
1 cup Peppermint Leaf
1 cup Chamomile Flowers
1 cup Thyme Leaf
1 cup Marshmallow Leaf
½ cup Wood Betony Leaf

"I allow my heart to be at peace"

HEMORRHOIDS

¼ cup Horse Chestnut Leaf
1 cup Bilberry Leaf
1 cup Chamomile Flowers
1 cup Plantain Leaf
1 cup Butchers Broom Leaf
Quart of Aloe Juice (non-acidic)
1 cup Horsetail Leaf
1 cup Dandelion Leaf
½ cup St John's Wort Leaf
1 cup Peppermint Leaf
1 cup Spearmint Leaf

"I am right on time to let go of the burdens of fear from the past."

HIGH CHOLESTEROL

1 cup Basil Leaf

1 cup Celery Seed

½ cup Fennel Seed

1 cup Parsley Leaf

½ cup Turmeric Root

1 cup Artichoke Leaf

1 cup Alfalfa Leaf

1 Whole Bulb Garlic

1 cup Echinacea Leaf

"I flow with the ever present joy of life."

HORMONAL BALANCE

1 cup Red Clover Leaf

1 cup Black Cohosh Leaf

1 cup Dong Quai Root

½ Licorice Root

1 cup Damiana Leaf

1 cup Vitex Leaf

¼ Hops Flowers

¼ Asian Ginseng Root

½ cup Ginkgo Leaf

½ cup Chaste Tree Leaf

1 cup False Unicorn Root

½ cup Sage Leaf

1 cup Raspberry Leaf

½ St John's Wort Leaf

1 cup Sarsaparilla Leaf

½ cup Saw Palmetto Berries

½ cup Shepard's Purse Leaf

½ cup True Unicorn Bark

¼ cup Wild Yam Bark

"I am restoring the proper balance to my life."

IMMUNE SYSTEM

½ cup Astragalus Root
½ cup Usnea Lichen
½ cup Sage Leaf
2 Juiced Bulbs of Garlic
½ cup Shitake Mushroom
½ cup Reishi Mushroom
1 cup Hyssop Leaf
1 cup St John's Wort Leaf
1 cup Bayberry Leaf
¼ cup Fenugreek Seeds ½
cup Dandelion Leaf
¼ cup Milk Thistle Seed
½ cup Ginseng Root
1 cup Echinacea Root
1 cup Echinacea Leaf
½ cup Licorice Root

"I am safe to now express and energize myself with joy!"

IMPOTENCE

1 cup Ginkgo Leaf
1 cup Yohimbe Bark
1 cup Panax Ginseng Root
1 cup Muira Puama Root
1 cup Damiana Leaf
½ cup Fo-ti Root
½ cup Tongkat Ali Root
¼ cup Maca Root
½ cup Horny Goat Weed
¼ cup Tribulus Leaf
½ cup False Unicorn Leaf
½ cup Guarana Leaf
¼ cup Ashwagandha Root
½ cup Saw Palmetto Berries
¼ cup Pygeum Bark

"I express generously through my sexual energy."

INCONTINENCE

1 cup Buchu Leaf
1 cup Saw Palmetto Berries
¼ cup Cardamom Seeds
1 cup Corn Silk
½ cup Dandelion Leaf
½ cup Horsetail Leaf
1 cup Lemon Balm Leaf
1 cup Spearmint Leaf
½ cup Juniper Berries
½ cup Uva Ursi Leaf

"I now decide to let go of controlling my emotions. I am in the flow."

IBS(Irritable Bowel Syndrome)

½ cup Milk Thistle Seed
Quart of Aloe Juice (non-acidic)
1 cup Alfalfa Leaf
1 cup Marshmallow Leaf
1 cup Slippery Elm Bark
1 cup Peppermint Leaf
¼ cup Asafetida Powder
1 cup Chamomile Flowers
½ cup Cramp Bark
½ cup Cascara Sagrada Bark

"I release old, decrepit ideas."

JAUNDICE

1 cup Dandelion Leaf
½ cup Silverweed
1 Quart Black Radish Juice
½ cup Milk Thistle Seed
1 cup Artichoke Leaf
1 cup St John's Wort Leaf
½ cup Blackthorn Tree
¼ cup Fennel Seeds
½ cup Nettles Leaf
¼ cup Horsetail Leaf
¼ cup Chamomile Flowers
¼ cup Angelica Root

"Everything I see is in Divine Order."

JOINTS

1 cup Alfalfa Leaf
1 cup Black Cohosh Leaf
1 cup Bladderwrack Leaf
¼ cup Oregano Leaf
3 tbl Cayenne Pepper 1
cup Celery Seed
1 cup Red Clover Leaf
½ cup Comfrey Root
½ cup Devils Claw Leaf
¼ cup Ginger Root
¼ cup Lemon Grass
½ cup Parsley Leaf
¼ cup Stinging Nettles Leaf
¼ cup Turmeric Root
¼ cup Burdock Root
¼ cup Chaparral Leaf
¼ cup Wild Yam
½ cup White Willow Bark

"I move through life flexible and with ease."

*Poultice and soaks may accompany tonic for optimal results.

KIDNEYS

1 cup Artichoke Leaf

¼ cup Birch Bark

½ cup Borage Leaf

1 cup Buchu Leaf

½ cup Dandelion Root

½ cup Siberian Ginseng

½ cup Fo-ti Root

1 cup Goldenrod Leaf

½ cup Gravel Root

½ cup Hydrangea Root

1 cup Uva Ursi Leaf

½ cup White Oak Bark

1 cup Parsley Leaf

½ cup Stinging Nettle Leaf

1 cup Yellow Dock Root

"I only look for good in every life situation."

LIVER

1 cup Dandelion Leaf
1 cup Milk Thistle Seeds
½ cup Oregon Grape Root
1 cup Burdock Root
1 cup Red Clover Leaf
1 cup Yellow Dock Leaf
½ cup Licorice Root
1 cup Celery Seed
1 cup Echinacea Leaf
1 cup Hyssop Leaf
½ cup Goldenseal Root
¼ cup Cayenne Pepper
1 cup Peppermint Leaf
½ cup Cascara Sagrada Bark
12 Squeezed Lemons

"I transform my anger into joy."

MALE WELL-BEING

1 cup Hawthorn Berries
1 cup Siberian Ginseng Root
½ cup American Ginseng Root
¼ cup Ginger Root
½ cup Ginkgo Root
½ cup Damiana Leaf
¼ cup Cinnamon Bark
¼ cup Horny Goat Weed
¼ cup Muira Puama Bark
½ cup Oat Straw
1 cup Sarsaparilla Bark
½ cup Saw Palmetto Berries
½ cup Yohimbe Bark
¼ cup Cordyceps Mushroom
¼ cup Reishi Mushroom
¼ cup Deer Antler

"I affirm only the best for my life"

MOTION SICKNESS

1 cup Holy Basil Leaf
½ cup Fennel Seed
1 cup Peppermint Leaf
½ cup Thyme Leaf
½ cup Anise Seed
½ cup Fennel Seed
½ cup Ginger Root
1 cup Chamomile Flowers

"I'm free."

MOUTH/GUMS

¼ cup Myrrh Gum

2 Quarts Aloe Juice (non-acidic)

½ cup Clove Bud

1 cup Neem Leaf

1 cup Calendula Flowers

1 cup Peppermint Leaf

¼ cup Spearmint Leaf 1

cup Sage Leaf

1 cup Echinacea Root

1 cup White Oak Bark

"I choose and support my own decisions."

NAUSEA

1 cup Anise Seed
¼ Fennel Seed
2 tbl Oregano Leaf
2 tbl Thyme
1 Bay Leaf
1 tsp Cayenne Pepper
1 cup Ginger Root
2 cups Peppermint Leaf
½ cup Goldenseal Leaf
3 tbl Nutmeg

"I have the courage to love beyond my fears."

*Also helps to sip slowly on ice water.

NERVES

1 cup Mullein Leaf
1 cup Sage Leaf
1 cup Elderberry
1 cup Slippery Elm Bark
1 Whole Bulb Garlic
1 ½ Echinacea Leaf
1 cup Yarrow Leaf
½ cup Ginger Root
1 cup Buchu Leaf
½ cup Goldenseal Root
½ cup Licorice Root
½ cup Lemon Balm Leaf
½ cup Oregano Leaf
½ cup Thyme Leaf

"I indulge in communication about how I feel."

NIGHT SWEATS

½ cup Dong Quai Root
¾ cup Black Cohosh Leaf
¼ cup Ginseng Root
½ cup Wild Yam Root
½ cup Red Clover Buds
½ cup Motherwort Leaf
½ cup Hops Flowers
¼ cup Sage Leaf
½ cup Vitex (Chaste Berries)
¼ cup Licorice Root
1 cup Alfalfa Leaf

"As anger rises to the surface, I gently release it."

NOSEBLEEDS

1 cup Bilberry Leaf
1 cup Nettle Leaf
¼ cup Cayenne Pepper
1 cup Raspberry Leaf
1 cup Witch Hazel Leaf
¼ cup Comfrey Root
½ cup Parsley Leaf
¼ cup Agrimony Leaf
¼ cup Yarrow Leaf

"I recognize and embrace the love I feel for me."

PMS

1 cup False Unicorn Root
1 cup Damiana Leaf
2 cups Red Raspberry Leaf
½ cup Fo-Ti Root
½ cup Wild Yam Root
½ cup Chasteberry (Vitex)
¼ cup Black Cohosh Leaf
½ cup Dong Quai Root
¼ cup St. John's Wort
¼ cup Burdock Root
¼ cup Lemon Balm Leaf
¼ cup Ginkgo Leaf
¼ cup Thyme Leaf
¼ cup Ginger Root
¼ cup Cinnamon Bark

"I am clear, powerful and satisfied with my feminine nature."

PAIN

1 cup Chamomile Leaf

¼ cup Clove Bud

1 cup Oat Straw

1 cup St John's Wort

½ cup Valerian Root

¼ cup Skullcap Leaf

½ cup Hops Flowers

1 cup Peppermint Leaf

1 cup Spearmint Leaf

½ cup Comfrey Root

¼ cup Kava Kava Root

¼ cup Ginger Root

½ cup Turmeric Powder

1 cup White Willow Bark

1 cup Hops Flowers

½ cup Cat's Claw Root

"ALL I thought I owed, is now paid up. I owe nothing."

PARASITES

1 cup Black Walnut
½ cup Cloves
1 cup Ginger Root
3 tbls Cayenne
¼ cup Golden Seal Root
½ cup Oregon Grape Root
1 cup Wormwood
½ cup Thyme Leaf
½ cup Barberry
½ cup Gentian Root
½ cup Oregano Leaf
Juice of Whole Bulb Garlic
Juice of Large Red Onion

"I have FULL power over my life."

PREGNANCY TEA

1 cup Spearmint Leaf

1 cup Raspberry Leaf

¾ cup Strawberry Leaf

1 cup Nettle Leaf

½ cup Rose Hips Fruit

¼ cup Fennel Seed

¼ cup Lemongrass Leaf

1 cup Alfalfa Leaf

½ cup Lemon Verbena Leaf

"I bring forth new life with grace and ease."

PROSTATE

1 cup Corn Silk
½ cup Bitter Melon Seeds
1 cup Raspberry Leaf
1 cup Plantain Leaf
1 cup Saw Palmetto Berries
½ cup Red Clover Leaf
½ cup Pygueum Bark
1 cup Stinging Nettles Leaf
1 cup Uva Ursi Leaf

"I am perfect in my imperfection."

RASHES

1 cup Calendula Flowers
½ cup Comfrey Root
1 cup Elder Flower
½ cup Red Clover Leaf
1 Quart Aloe Juice (non-acidic)
½ cup Milk Thistle Seeds
1 cup Dandelion Leaf
½ cup Burdock Root
1 cup Alfalfa Leaf
1 cup Yellow Dock Leaf

"I am patient with the processes of life."

SCALP ISSUES

1 cup Rosemary Leaf
1 cup Nettles Leaf
½ cup Burdock Root
¼ cup Turmeric Root
½ cup Ginger Root
1 cup Sarsaparilla Root
½ cup Figwort Leaf
½ cup Oregon Grape Root
½ cup Yellow Dock Leaf
¼ cup Valerian Root
½ cup Skullcap Leaf

"I am crowned with glory and honor."

SCARS

2 Quarts Aloe Juice (non-acidic)
½ cup Comfrey Root
½ cup Black Walnut Leaf
1 cup Chamomile Flowers
1 cup Calendula Flowers
¼ cup Lavender Flowers

"I forgive and let it go."

SEXUAL ORGANS

1 cup Ginseng Root
½ cup Cardamom Seed
3 tsp Nutmeg
½ cup Muira Puama
½ cup Horny Goat Weed
1 cup Fo-ti Root
1 cup Damania Leaf
½ cup Maca Root
½ cup Yohimbe Bark
1 cup Passionflower

"I am full of amazing, satisfying and powerful creative energy"

SINUS

1 cup Eucalyptus Leaf
¼ cup Licorice Root
¼ cup Horseradish Root grated
½ cup Nettle Leaf
1 cup Peppermint Leaf
½ cup Ginger Root grated
½ cup Echinacea Root
¼ cup Golden Seal Root
1 cup Elder Berry
½ cup Fenugreek Seed
½ cup Thyme Leaf
¼ cup Juniper Berries
½ cup Calendula Flowers
¼ cup Myrrh Bark
1 tablespoon Cayenne Pepper (or to taste)

"I am agreeable with all those around me."

STOMACH

1 cup Buchu Leaf
½ cup Fennel Seed
½ cup Ginger Root
1 cup Marshmallow Leaf
1 cup Slippery Elm Bark
1 cup Anise Seed
¼ cup Caraway Seed

"I effortlessly digest my life, just as it is."

THROAT

1 cup Peppermint Leaf
½ Spearmint Leaf
½ cup Ginger Root
½ cup Slippery Elm Bark
½ cup Licorice Root
½ cup Marshmallow Root
½ cup Honeysuckle Flowers
1 cup Horehound Leaf
¼ cup Sage Leaf
LOTS OF RAW HONEY!

"I speak only my truth with love and sweetness."

*Additional Note:
Horehound Syrup can be used here for those who cannot tolerate certain sweeteners.
Ingredients:
½ cup horehound (flowering tops), 1 cup hot water, 2 cups local raw honey (adjust to taste)

THYROID

1 cup Echinacea Leaf
¼ cup Licorice Root
¼ cup Bugleweed Leaf
½ cup Siberian Ginseng Root
½ cup Bladderwrack Leaf
¼ cup Black Walnut Leaf
½ cup Lemon Balm
¼ Ashwagandha Root
½ cup Schizandra Berries

"I am regenerating right now."

TONSILLITIS

1 cup White Oak Bark
1 cup Witch Hazel Leaf
½ cup White Willow Bark
½ cup St. John's Wort
1 cup Goldenseal Leaf
1 cup Echinacea Leaf
1 cup Raspberry Leaf
1 cup Pau d'Arco

"I freely express my creativity."

TORN LIGAMENTS

1 cup Horsetail Leaf

1 cup Devils Claw Root

1   cup Comfrey Root

2   Quarts Aloe Juice (non-acidic)

1 cup Peppermint Leaf

1 cup Pennywort Leaf

"I am allowing my life to be restored."

URINARY INFECTION

1 cup Celery Seed
½ cup Fennel Seed
2 cups Corn Silk
2 cups Parsley Leaf
1 cup Spearmint Leaf
1 Quart Pure Cranberry Juice
½ cup Horseradish grated
1 cup Marshmallow Leaf
¼ cup Uva Ursi Leaf
¼ cup Horsetail Leaf
¼ cup Dandelion Root
¼ cup Yellow Root
1 cup Echinacea Leaf
½ cup Nettles Leaf

"Life is a sheer delight and I am happy with my life partners."

VARICOSE VEINS

½ cup Horse Chestnut Leaf
½ cup Gotu Kola Leaf
1 cup Butchers Broom leaf
1 cup Witch Hazel Leaf
1 cup Violet Leaf
1 cup Calendula Flowers
1 cup Ginger Root
1 cup Ginkgo Leaf
¼ cup Cayenne Pepper
1 cup Rosemary Leaf
1 cup Yarrow Leaf
1 cup Hawthorn Berries

"I flow with the currency of gratitude."

*Poultices and baths can also be used for effectiveness.

WEIGHT LOSS

1 cup Sarsaparilla Bark

¼ cup Licorice Root

1 cup Corn Silk

¼ cup Horehound Leaf

½ cup Kelp

½ cup Bladderwrack

½ cup Echinacea Leaf

1 cup Chickweed Leaf

¼ cup Burdock Root

¼ cup Black Walnut Hulls

1 cup Cleavers Leaf

½ cup Yerba Mate Leaf

½ cup Plantain Leaf

1 cup Spearmint Leaf

½ cup Oat Straw

"I allow others to align with the goodness that I am."

ABOUT THE AUTHOR

Since 1988, Ombassa Sophera has combined years of herbal study, a legacy of home remedies, and wellness coaching, to provide viable solutions to leading rich, holistic and enriching lives.

In 1993, she founded The Natural Healers Network, a health event series for health and wellness practitioners in Atlanta, GA, which included: organic cooking courses, reiki, iridology and a host of other alternative health modalities. In 1997, she began facilitating her signature workshop entitled, "Taking Responsibility for Your Health and Well-Being"

Ombassa is dedicated to assisting humanity to awaken to its ultimate potential, dreams and aspirations. Her work encompasses balancing WHOLE BODY SYSTEMS, guiding you towards ultimate health from the inside-out, while creating new and improved blueprints for living your passion and purpose.

Ombassa's philosophy: "while stress consistently has a stronghold on people's lives–causing; debilitating illnesses, relationship breakups, unhappiness and depression, the key to healing isn't just ingesting an anecdote of any sort, more importantly, it is to purge yourself of the thoughts and emotions that make these imbalances possible".

Also an Intuitive healer, who uses her innate gifts to scan clients energy body to identify imbalances within, she is able to pinpoint the underlining dis-ease and assist her client to heal the body, mind and spirit.

She has authored three books—Soul Journey to Truth, Inspire Yourself and ABC's of Nature's Best Herbal Recipes, two meditation CDs—SolJoy in Love and Soul Journey to Truth, Ombassa also provides custom herbal consultations through her blog and conducts workshops on herbal medicine, mindfulness and self-love across the USA and abroad.

She is co-founder of Life Conversations Radio and Host of The P.L.A.Y. (Passionately Loving Appreciating YOU!) Experience.

www.ombassa.com

LIST OF HERBAL SUPPLIERS

Starwest Botanicals
www.starwest-botanicals.com

Herbco
www.herbco.com/Wholesale-Herbs

Atlantic Spice
www.atlanticspice.com

Traditional Medicinals
www.traditionalmedicinals.com

Frontier Coop
www.frontiercoop.com

Mountain Rose
www.mountainroseherbs.com

Taos Herb
www.taosherb.com